Combating Eating Disorders

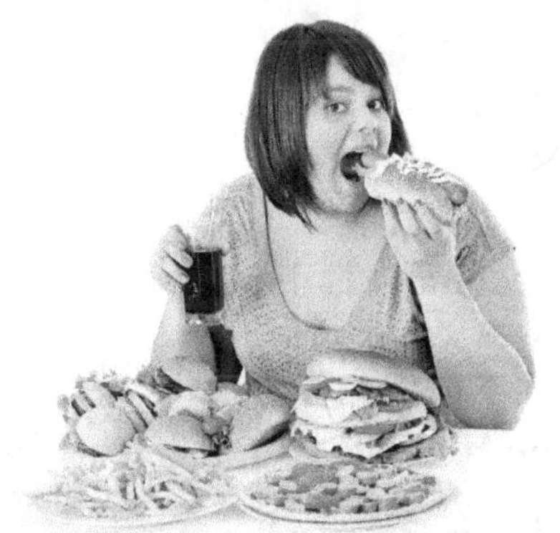

How to get over Binge Eating, Bulimia Nervosa, and Anorexia Nervosa

Victoria Simeon

TABLE OF CONTENT

Introduction:

Do you eat in unusually large quantities or until you feel stuffed?

Do you think your eating habits are beyond your control?

Have you attempted weight loss? How, then?

Do you ever eat ostentatiously?

Are you depressed, embarrassed, or guilty about what you eat? Do you worry about your weight in any way?

Have you ever gone to the bathroom to burn calories?

My aunt once had an eating disorder (Bulimia Nervosa) which made everyone in the home develop a fear of eating.

We started engaging in different exercises to lose weight which eventually led to my sister developing anorexia. So this was me having two members of my family with similar problems caused by overeating and under-eating. I became confused not knowing whose steps to follow, my aunt's or my sister?

Eventually, we were able to help my aunt scale through her binge dieting not by avoiding what she likes. Now she appreciates her body image and is self confident. while my sister is back on her feet ready to live a life of rediscovery.

This book will help you understand binge eating disorders like bulimia and anorexia Nervosa and how to overcome them and also give you a good perception of your body image.

Join me as we embark on a path to Eliminating Binge eating disorders and living a healthy life…

1.

Binge Eating

Binge eating is a type of disordered eating that involves eating uncontrollably for extended periods. It is a common symptom of eating disorders like bulimia nervosa and binge eating disorder.

A person quickly consumes an excessive amount of food during such binges. Feelings of being out of control are linked to a diagnosis of binge eating.

When you feel like you can't stop eating and consistently consume large amounts of food, you are experiencing a significant eating disorder called a binge.

Nearly everybody indulges once in a while, for example, having seconds or thirds of a vacation dinner.

However, for some people, binge-eating disorder crosses the line when excessive overeating that feels out of control becomes a regular occurrence.

At the point when you have a voraciously consuming food problem, you might be humiliated about indulging and commit to stopping. However,you are so compelled that you are unable to resist the urges and continue your binge eating.

Being overweight and obese are also linked to binge eating disorder. This is more likely to affect women than men. Although binge eating disorder can affect people of any age, it typically manifests in the late teens or early twenties.

Factors that can lead to Eating disorders are:

Family history of eating disorders, depression, addiction to alcohol or drugs; have been bullied or criticized for your eating habits, body shape, or weight; are overly concerned with being slim; suffer from anxiety, low self-esteem, an obsessive personality, or are a perfectionist; or have been sexually abused.

Like other eating disorders, binge eating disorder is caused by a combination of genetics, thoughts, and feelings, especially about one's weight and body shape, cultural and social issues, and one's surroundings.

Dieting in unhealthy ways, like skipping meals, not eating enough, or avoiding certain foods, may lead to binge eating for some people.

The Symptoms

The majority of people who suffer from binge-eating disorders are obese or overweight, but you might be a normal weight. The emotional and behavioral signs of binge eating disorder include:

•Consuming food to an uncomfortably full extent.

•Eating a lot of food in a short time, like two hours, in an unusually large amount.

•Having the impression that your eating habits are out of control.

•Frequently eating by themselves or in private.

•Eating despite feeling full or hungry.

•Consuming food quickly during binge periods.

•Experiencing feelings of depression, disgust, shame, guilt, or anger regarding your eating.

•Going on frequent diets, which may or may not result in weight loss.

Unlike with bulimia, you don't always use laxatives, exercise too much, or vomit after a binge to make up for the extra calories you ate. You can try to eat normally or go on a diet.

However, restricting your diet may only result in more binges.

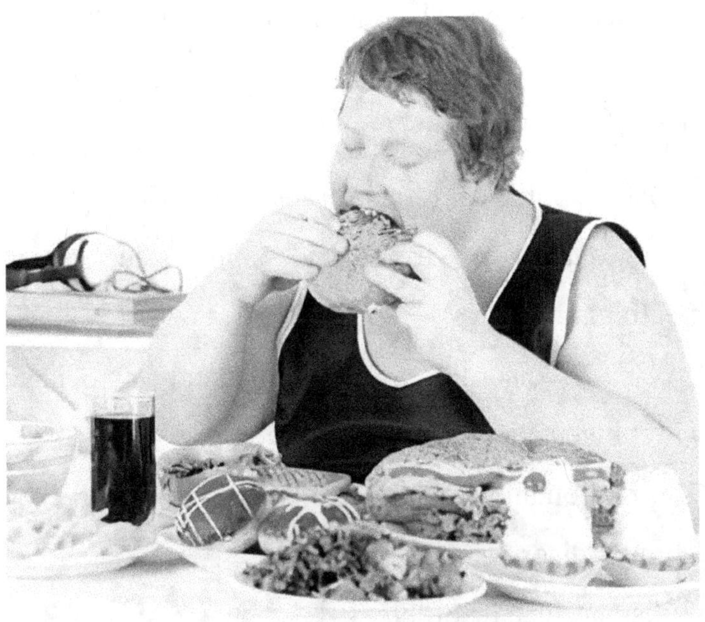

It's Complications:

You may experience mental and physical issues as a result of binge eating. These issues may be caused by binge-eating disorder

•Obesity or medical conditions related to obesity, such as joint problems, heart disease, type 2 diabetes.

• Gastroesophageal reflux disease (GERD).

•Poor quality of life and some sleep-related breathing disorders.

Psychiatric disorders that are frequently associated with binge eating disorder include:

•Depression and Anxiety

•Bipolar disorder

•Substance use disorders.

2.

Bulimia Nervosa

Bulimia Nervosa, more commonly known as bulimia, is a serious eating disorder with the potential to endanger one's life. Bulimia sufferers may secretly binge, consuming large quantities of food while losing control, and then purge, attempting to lose calories in an unhealthy way.

It is characterized by binge-like cycles with compensatory behaviors. Any behavior that serves to "make up for" the binge is compensatory behavior.
Examples of these behaviors include fasting, obsessive exercise, abuse of laxatives, and self-induced vomiting.

It Is a common misunderstanding that an individual with an eating disorder can be identified by their appearance alone. This is false because many people who suffer from bulimia may be of average weight or have larger bodies.

Identifying the signs that you or a loved one may be experiencing the physical side effects of bulimia can be made easier if you are aware of them.

Physical Symptoms of Bulimia In the early stages of an eating disorder

You might not exhibit many symptoms. They may be mild if you do. Some physical side effects in the short term are:

Electrolyte imbalances, Anemia, Fatigue, Sore throat, Stomach pain, Bloating,

Blood sugar fluctuations, Bacterial infections, Feeling full after eating only small amounts, Constipation, Irregular heart rhythm, Amenorrhea also known as the absence of menstruation, Cavities, Swollen salivary glands in the jaw or neck, Hair loss, Dry skin, Yellow-orange skin, Sleep problems, Dizziness, Pancreatitis.

Every bodily system can be impacted by bulimia. Since most individuals with bulimia gorge then vomit, most examination centers around the effect of drawn-out self-actuated regurgitating.

Other disordered eating behaviors, such as excessive laxative use, compulsive exercise, and food restriction, are common among those with bulimia. These actions may result in their symptoms.

Bulimia can have several long-term effects, including: Fertility issues, Type 2 diabetes, Kidney damage Increased risk of kidney stones and kidney failure Damaged nerve endings in the bowel, Weakness in the esophageal sphincter, Tearing of the esophagus, Ulcers, lining of the intestines, Chronic acid reflux Esophagitis, an inflammation of the esophagus that can lead to scarring Esophageal cancer Ruptured esophagus or stomach due to binging and purging.

3.

Anorexia Nervosa

Anorexia nervosa is a serious eating disorder that can lead to death but can be treated. Extreme food restrictions and a strong fear of gaining weight are its hallmarks. Individuals with anorexia limit the number of calories and the kinds of food they eat.

They eventually lose weight or are unable to maintain a healthy weight for their height, age, stature, and overall health. They might exercise obsessively, purge the food they eat, misuse laxatives or intentionally vomit.

Anorexics also have a negative self-image of their bodies and a strong fear of gaining weight.

Anorexics who lose a lot of weight can become malnourished, have dangerous health issues, or even die. Psychological therapy, nutritional counseling, and hospitalization are typical components of treatment.

Anorexia can affect people of any age, sex, gender, race, ethnicity, sexual orientation, or economic status. It can also affect people of any size, weight,
or shape.

Anorexia is most common in young women and adolescents, but it also affects men and is becoming more common in children and older adults.

What symptoms does anorexia present?

Because anorexia involves mental and behavioral aspects in addition to physical ones, it is impossible to diagnose anorexia solely based on a person's physical appearance.

An individual needn't bother with being underweight to have anorexia. Anorexia can also affect people who have larger bodies.

However, cultural prejudice against fat and obesity may make it less likely that they will be diagnosed. Additionally, being underweight can occur without anorexia.

Keep in mind that in addition to its physical manifestations, anorexia also has psychological and behavioral aspects.

Anorexia is characterized by several physical, emotional, and behavioral signs and symptoms. It is essential to seek assistance if you or someone you know exhibits the following signs and symptoms of anorexia.

•Being extremely afraid of gaining weight.

•Having a distorted self-image and being unable to evaluate your body shape and weight in a realistic manner.

•Having an insatiable interest in diets, calories, and food.

•Being very critical of oneself.

•Feeling a powerful urge to be in charge.

•Irritability or depression.

•Having suicidal or self-harming thoughts.

•Changes in eating routines or habits, such as rearranging food on a plate or cutting out particular food groups or types.

•Despite losing weight, making frequent remarks about feeling "fat" or overweight.

•Using laxatives or diuretics improperly, intentionally vomiting, or going to the bathroom right after eating.

•Utilizing appetite suppressants or diet pills.

•Excessive and obsessive physical activity or intense physical training.

•Maintaining a diet even when your weight is below average for your height, stature, and sex.

• Making food for other people but not for oneself.

•Wearing a free dress or potentially wearing layers to conceal weight reduction and remain warm.

•Removing oneself from social gatherings and friends.

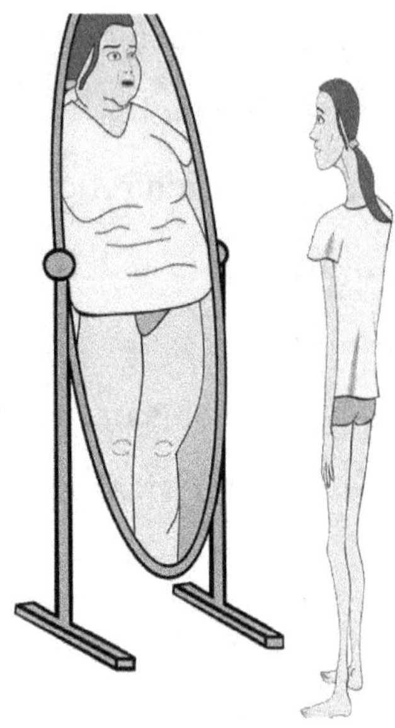

Anorexia's physical signs and symptoms include:

Being underweight for one's height, sex, and stature, which is the most well-known physical sign. However, it is essential to keep in mind that anorexia can occur in people who are overweight.

Physical signs of anorexia that are side effects of starvation and malnutrition exist alongside the weight-related symptoms.

Anorexia-like symptoms include:
•Substantial weight loss for several weeks or months.
•Not keeping a weight that is right for your height, age, sex, stature, and overall health.
•Changes in the growth curve or body mass index (BMI) are not explained in children and adolescents who are still growing.
The following are physical symptoms of anorexia that are brought on by starvation and malnutrition:
•Fainting, dizziness or being worn out.
•Heartbeat that is either irregular or slow.
•Hypotension or low blood pressure,
•Inability to concentrate and focus.
•Being constantly cold.

•Amenorrhea or irregular menstruation

•Difficulty in breathing.

•Abdominal pain or bloating.

•Loss of muscle mass and muscle weakness.

•Brittle nails, dry skin, and/or thinning hair.

•Infrequent illness and inadequate wound healing.

•The hands and feet are colored purple or bluish-purple.

Difference between Anorexia Nervosa and Bulimia Nervosa

Eating disorders include bulimia nervosa and anorexia nervosa. They may exhibit similar symptoms, such as an intense fear of gaining weight and a negative body image. Their distinct food-related behaviors are different.

To lose weight, people with anorexia drastically cut calories and/or purge.

Individuals who have bulimia eat an extreme measure of food in a brief timeframe (pigging out) trailed by specific ways of behaving to forestall weight gain. These actions include:

•Deliberate (self-actuated) spewing.
•Misuse of medications like thyroid hormones or laxatives.
•Excessive exercise or fasting.

When someone has anorexia, they typically have a body mass index (BMI) of less than 18.455 kg/m2 (kilograms per square body), especially if they have a physical disability.

ANOREXIA AFFECTS

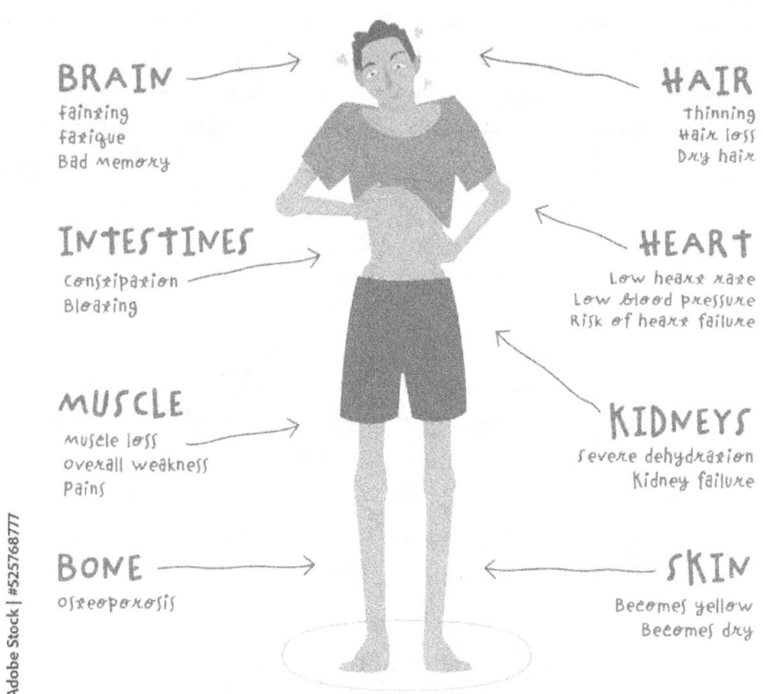

Adobe Stock | #525768777

4.

Fight against Anorexia

If you fall into the hands of anorexia after suffering from bulimia or trying to prevent it, thinking you might never experience an eating disorder again, don't take it as a big deal; instead, fight against it.

The good news is that you can unlearn the behaviors you've acquired. You can always overcome through determination. Anyone can get better, just as anyone can develop an eating disorder.

However, there is more to overcoming an eating disorder than just giving up bad eating habits.

In addition, it involves developing new strategies for coping with emotional pain and rediscovering who you are beyond your eating habits, weight, and body image.

To Deal with this you need to:
•know the causes first.
•Take a break (don't worry too much, it will only make things worse).
•Buy foods you like.
•Practice smart eating (add extras to your dishes, eat more red meat, pork, and fatty foods).
•Watch what you drink, especially before eating.
•Exercise (you can build muscle to gain weight).

5.

Your Body Image

The way we perceive our physical appearance and our thoughts and feelings about it are referred to as our body image.

There are numerous ways to think about our bodies and appearance when discussing body image. You might discover that there are times when you are unhappy with your appearance and other times when you like parts of your body.

Your weight is only one aspect of body image; other factors include:

•Finding it difficult to find clothes for your body, especially if you have a physical disability.

•Having the impression that people don't understand your body when they assume things like why you might require a wheelchair.

•Feeling like you are not attractive enough Birthmarks, surgery scars, or acne affecting how you feel about how you look.

•Sensing that your appearance does not correspond to your gender.

If you're having these thoughts and feelings about how you look, it could be that you're having trouble with your body image.

You might find regular errands like eating, getting dressed, or going out with companions turning out to be more troublesome.

This can happen at any time or consistently throughout your life, but it's common to think like this during puberty. Your body releases hormones during puberty that make you more aware of how you look and of other people's bodies.

Everybody experiences these changes, which can occasionally make you feel out of control or anxious.

It can also make you feel Low confident, Despondent, Uneasy, Confined and dejected, you start developing eating issues, or fixating on what you look like.

What to do assuming you are fixated (obsessed) on your look.

It is essential to keep in mind that there is no one type of beauty, Everyone has a unique perspective on it. Additionally, there is no right or wrong approach.

However, if you're having trouble, the following steps can be taken:

•Do whatever it takes not to contrast yourself with the many pictures you see on the web and in magazines, which are frequently carefully different to make them look awesome.

•Concentrate on the positive aspects of yourself and your body that you find appealing.

•Spend time with people who make you feel good about who you are. It might be helpful to write down the nice things people say to you, not just about how you look. Keep in mind that there are numerous reasons why people value you.

•What advice would you give a friend? When you start to have negative thoughts, keep in mind the piece of advice you would give to a friend if they told you they were having trouble with their appearance.

•Talk to someone you can rely on, like your parents or other members of your extended family, like older cousins, aunts, or uncles. It could be a neighbor, a teacher, a close family member, or someone from a club you belong to outside of your home.

•Be thoughtful of yourself.

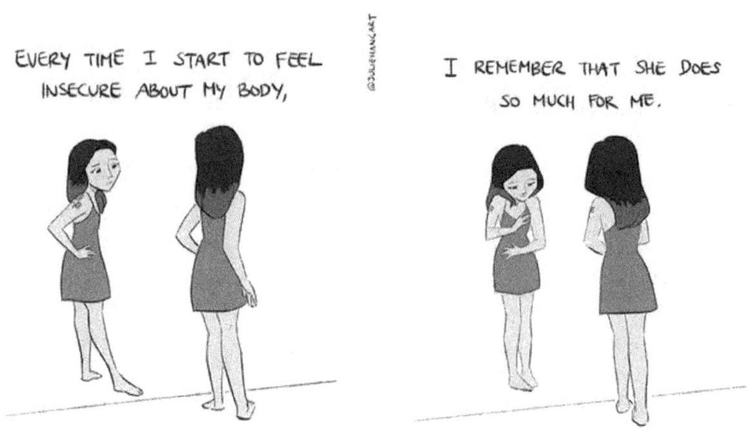

" Behind what you see, you are so much more. You are distinctive in every way imaginable. Nobody else has your experiences, passion, way of life, smile, or heart and soul as you do. You are unique. This merits celebration because, ultimately, true beauty does not depend on how you look. It has to do with who you are as a person and how you make other people feel about themselves."

6.

Support and coping strategies

Living with an eating disorder is particularly challenging because you have to deal with food every day. To help you cope, here are some suggestions:

•Consume breakfast: Breakfast is skipped by many people with binge eating disorders. However, if you eat breakfast, you might be less likely to eat meals later in the day that have more calories.

•Dieting should be avoided unless supervised. If you try to lose weight, you might have more binge-like episodes, which can be hard to break.

Talk to your doctor about the best ways to manage your eating disorder. You shouldn't diet unless it's recommended by your doctor and under his or her supervision.

•Get the nutrients you need: During binges, just because you eat a lot doesn't mean you're getting all the necessary nutrients from the food you're eating. If you need to change your diet to get the necessary vitamins and minerals, ask your doctor.

•Set up your surroundings: For some people, the availability of particular foods can lead to binges. Limit your exposure to foods that can lead to binge eating or keep them out of your home as much as possible.

•Maintain contact: Don't shut yourself off from supportive friends and family who want to see you get healthy. Recognize that they are thinking about your best interests.

•Get moving: If you have health issues related to being overweight, talk to your doctor about what kind of physical activity would be best for you.

•Alternative medicine: The majority of herbal supplements and dietary supplements that claim to help people lose weight or suppress their appetite are ineffective and may be misused by people with eating disorders.

Herbs and supplements for weight loss may interact dangerously with other medications and cause serious side effects. If you take herbs or dietary supplements, talk to your doctor to know about the possible side effects .

•Be gentle with yourself, Don't give in to your self-doubt.

•Search for positive good examples who can assist with lifting your confidence. Keep in mind that the thin models and actresses featured in women's magazines often don't have healthy bodies.

•Try to locate a trusted friend or relative with whom you can discuss the situation.

•Try to find a partner in the fight against binge eating, someone you can turn to for support rather than food.

•Track down solid ways of sustaining yourself by helping fun or to unwind, like yoga, contemplation, or just a walk.

•Write down your thoughts, feelings, and actions in a journal. Journaling can help you become more aware of the connections between your actions and feelings.

•Get support If you suffer from a binge-eating disorder, you and your loved ones may find that joining support groups provides you with support, hope, and strategies for coping.

Because they have been through what you are going through, members of your support group can empathize with you.

Find out if your doctor or nurse knows of a group in your area.

•Get ready for your appointment: The treatment of binge eating disorder may necessitate a team effort that includes dietitians with experience in eating disorders, mental health professionals, and other medical professionals.

You can use this information to prepare for your appointments. Make a list of these things before your appointment:

Key personal information, such as any major stresses or recent life changes, as well as the dosages of any herbs, vitamins, or other supplements you take, as well as any medications you are taking.

A typical day's eating, which can help your medical care provider or mental health professional to understand your eating habits.

Questions to ask your medical care provider or mental health professional include:

•What medicines are accessible, and which do you suggest?

•Is there a generic medication available if medication is part of the treatment?

•Can I obtain any printed materials, such as brochures? Which websites do you suggest?

During your appointment, don't be shy about asking any additional questions.

7.

Fad Diets

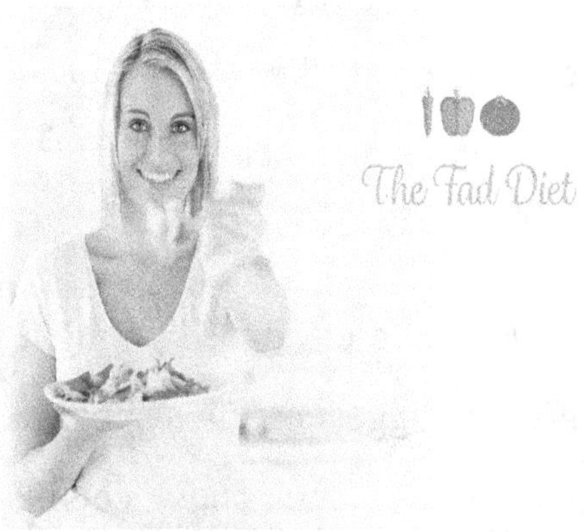

Fad diets are diet plans which promise quick weight loss but lack solid scientific evidence to back up its claims. Plans that require you to eat very few foods or unusual combinations of foods are common. You might only be able to eat certain foods at specific times.

Fad diets frequently include expensive and unnecessary food ingredients, supplements, and/or food products.

This cycle can have an impact on our relationship with food, resulting in feelings of failure rather than the development of the skills and self-assurance necessary to maintain a healthy diet and weight.

Some popular fad diets are : Banning a specific food or food group; suggest eating a specific food or food group only to change body chemistry; suggest hormone changes as the cause of weight gain and attempt to change it.

•Diets with a lot of protein, fat, and carbs are often low in calcium, fiber, and plant proteins.

The Grapefruit diet and The South Beach Diet are two examples.

Yogurt, cheese, milk, and ice cream White bread, white pasta, and white rice Foods made with refined white flour, like pancakes and bagels Low-fiber cereal, either hot or cold Canned vegetables Fresh vegetables in small amounts if they are well-cooked, Potatoes without the skin, Eggs Dairy products if your body can process them well, Tender protein sources, like eggs, tofu, chicken, and fish Creamy peanut butter, Fats, like olive oil, mayonnaise.

•Diets high in carbohydrates and fiber but low in protein, such as those made with peas, apples, bananas, tomatoes, broccoli, legumes, coconut oil, and avocados.

Here Is an in-depth look at seven well-liked approaches to dieting and weight loss:

1. Juice fasts and diets are a great way to "reset" your body in preparation for a more long-term weight loss plan. In the long run, replacing a meal with juice is perfectly safe and healthy.

However, instead of extracting juice, try blending whole fruits and vegetables into a smoothie or adding fiber-rich foods to help prevent hunger. Juice diets can range from replacing one meal with juice (typically made from a combination of fresh fruits and vegetables) to eliminating calories.

2. Current research indicates that intermittent fasting is a legitimate and risk-free method of weight loss.
If you decide to try intermittent fasting for the first time, start with a less strict program like the 16/8 method and work your way up to something more extreme like alternate-day fasting. Some even let you fast if your lifestyle allows it.

However, regulate your relationship with food with caution. Stop the diet if, at any point, you begin to engage in risky behaviors like binging and purging or restricting food for longer than the program allows.

3. The Paleo and keto diets' suggestions: The Paleo and keto diets have many universally beneficial tenets.

High-quality carbs, avoiding processed foods and refined grains, eating more leafy vegetables, and limiting or eliminating all refined sugar are all things that should be considered by everyone.

Spaghetti squash, sweet potatoes, riced cauliflower, and brown rice can take the place of carbs like pasta and white rice.

Be aware that once you stop following these diets, the weight will come back on.

Before beginning the keto diet, you should read this if you are an avid lifter.

4. Cutting carbs: In general, it's a good idea to cut back on carbs. Cutting back on carbohydrates can be a good thing.

However, before eliminating carbs, concentrate on getting the best carbs you can. All of the vitamins and fiber that carbs provide in terms of nutrition are eliminated by refined carbohydrates. Choose whole-wheat bread and pasta instead.

Start substituting vegetables like butternut squash, sweet potato, riced broccoli, and cauliflower for rice and pasta if you are willing to take the next step. Consume carbs like millet, brown rice, bulgur, quinoa, and brown rice, which are much more slowly absorbed than refined grains.

5. Teas for weight loss.

6. Consume high-calorie shakes or smoothies For people who don't eat much, a high-calorie shake or smoothie may be more appealing than a substantial meal.

These give you calories that are high in nutrients without making you feel too full. The following can be included in nutritious smoothies: Fruits, nuts, seeds, and greens like spinach.

7. The grapefruit and cabbage soup diets.

Can Dieting Stop Eating Disorders?

Fad dieting is a good way to recover from Bulimia but for some, fad dieting is simply a diet. Even people who regularly follow fad diets are unlikely to develop an eating disorder.

However, for some, fad dieting is the beginning of a much larger problem. It can be challenging to determine whether a real problem exists because it can be difficult to distinguish between true disordered eating behaviors and fad diets.

Fad diets can be appealing to people who are interested in losing weight or improving their physical appearance. Many of these diets guarantee remarkable effects within a short period of time.

Fad diets require dieters to engage in risky behaviors, such as eliminating entire food groups, fasting for extended periods, or drastically reducing overall food intake, to achieve these outcomes.

Dieters run the risk of developing an eating disorder by engaging in each of these actions.

To keep a healthy weight over the long term, balanced, therapeutic behavioral nutrition, behavior modification, individualized meal planning, understanding of the causes of emotions that arise around food, and Changes that last a lifetime are what will keep you healthy for the rest of your life.

The basic problem with many fad diets is that it's hard to maintain them for weeks, months, or even years. Which is not safe for one's health.

A lot of fad diets set the stage by cutting out entire food groups. This is a surefire way to fail. Keto demands you ought to stay away from bread, pasta, and rice no matter what. Paleo requires you to eliminate foods that cannot be gathered or hunted. Raw food diets convince you that cooking removes most of the nutrients from your food.

In addition, cutting things into pieces does not foster a healthy relationship with food.Rather, it spreads the false idea that some foods are either "good" or "bad".

It forces every food into one category or another, elevating some foods to pedestals and instilling guilt and shame in others. The way foods work is seriously oversimplified in this. Of course, it's not the smartest plan to have pizza all week long or eat a whole bundle of desserts in a solitary sitting.

However, you won't immediately be harmed if you incorporate these highly palatable foods into a comprehensive nutritional strategy.

Problems develop when you consume too much of any one thing. Having a bite of cake or small scoops of ice cream isn't a bad idea.

Packing food sources into one box or the other is a more destructive way to deal with nourishment than eating the food sources themselves. After all, you can overeat salads, nuts, avocados, granola, and salads. Fad diets, especially those with strict restrictions, are best avoided to avoid developing eating disorders.

Focusing on eating a healthy, well-balanced diet is preferable to obsessing over calories, specific food groups, or macronutrients.

People can maintain a healthy weight by eating enough calories and getting enough nutrients.

If a person is overweight and needs to lose a few pounds, they should only make changes to their diet and physical activity when a doctor tells them to.

Fad diets can lead to anorexia because many of them encourage eating very little food each day. They often require a person to cut out a portion of food, like carbohydrates, that may be abundant in their diet.

What works if dieting doesn't?

Restrictions and deprivation are ineffective! Instead of counting calories, it's more about the QUALITY OF THE CALORIES!

Diets simply do not meet the nutritional needs of each person based on age, sex, and ethnicity, as well as emotional eating needs (for food satisfaction). If you don't like what you're eating, you won't stick with it! Therefore, instead of focusing on calories, prioritize food quality. Scaling back calories, the revered way to deal with weight reduction will work for the present moment.

However, the body responds to calorie restriction in predictable ways by increasing hunger, slowing metabolic rate, and producing stress hormones, so this seemingly straightforward approach ultimately fails for the majority of people.

A well-balanced diet that focuses more on whole foods (vegetables, fruits, unprocessed grains, high-quality protein, and natural fats) is effective. In their natural state, whole foods are slowly digested, resulting in a steady rise in blood sugar without spikes or crashes. Blood sugar, hormones, and insulin change more slowly after a meal when you eat this way. Fat cells become calmer and store less fat. Hunger goes down. The metabolic rate rises. Without restriction or deprivation, this is a recipe for maintaining weight control over time.

To accomplish this normal, sound approach to eating,

First, stick to whole, high-quality fruits, vegetables, legumes, and small amounts of whole-kernel grains instead of processed carbs.

Second, consume sufficient quantities of high-quality protein, which includes plant proteins.

Third, indulge in high-fat foods like olive oil, nuts, and nut butter because fat is filling and has little effect on insulin. Quality matters once more!

Stay with something that can last for a long time when it comes to nutrition.

To get good healthy and nutritious recipes that are easy to make and can help you overcome binge eating get my book:

HEALTHY EATING COOKBOOK

A 21-Day Meal Plan for Weight Loss and Binge Eating recovery,

+20 Extra Recipes

By Victoria Simeon

CLICK HERE TO GET THE HEALTHY EATING COOKBOOK

 Understanding that your requirements determine an approach to nutrition that is sustainable for you .

"The best diet Is simply a lifestyle that includes eating what you like, exercising, and having healthy habits. Practicing mindful eating and exercise. Incorporating regular physical activity into your daily life."

8.

Recovery

Recovery does not mean that you will never have an eating disorder again. It entails not allowing it to dictate your life. It entails acknowledging your beauty and value despite all the time you've spent thinking otherwise.

Admitting you have an eating disorder is the first step toward recovery. This admission can be difficult, especially if you still believe, even subconsciously, that losing weight is the key to happiness, confidence, and success. Even when you finally realize that this isn't true, it can be hard to break old habits.

Accepting that you have an eating disorder and accepting yourself for the brave, strong, and magnificent person you are because you have learned to fight for yourself and overcome that obstacle is what this means.

It entails taking care of your body and maintaining its health because you deserve to be loved for who you are. It entails not giving in when faced with a fallback, even though you are aware that it is only one of a million steps forward. Recognizing that fighting is not the same as losing.

Anorexia and bulimia inner voices tell you that your worth is determined by how you look and that you will never be happy until you lose weight. Bliss and confidence come from adoring yourself for who you genuinely are — and that is just conceivable with recuperation.

Learning to overcome an eating disorder requires learning to:
•Listen to how you feel.
•Follow your body's cues.
•Accept who you are.
•Love yourself.

In Conclusion

It is possible to fully recover. A self-fulfilling prophecy can occur when you begin to lose hope.

Maintain a positive outlook and contact your therapist whenever you notice emotional difficulties. Although this may seem like a lot to deal with, keep in mind that you are not alone.

The path to recovery Is open to you, and help is readily available. With the correct guidance and support, you can overcome the negative patterns that your eating disorder has induced, reclaim your health, and rediscover your joy in life.